CAPTURED

CAPTURED

Mental and Physical Health Challenges

TRACY STEADMAN HENRY

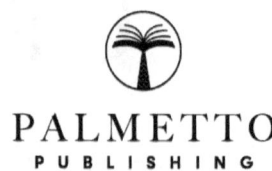

PALMETTO
P U B L I S H I N G
Charleston, SC
www.PalmettoPublishing.com

Copyright © 2024 by Tracy Steadman Henry

All rights reserved

No portion of this book may be reproduced, stored in a retrieval system, or transmitted in any form by any means–electronic, mechanical, photocopy, recording, or other–except for brief quotations in printed reviews, without prior permission of the author.

Paperback ISBN: 979-8-8229-4459-6

Dedication

To my therapist, JJ, without whom I wouldn't have been able to write this book.

To all who suffer from PTSD, trauma, anxiety, depression, and various other challenges, there is a light at the end of the tunnel. Acknowledge the past, try to live in the present, and tell your stories so they won't be forgotten in the future.

To my grandma and grandpa:
I will forever love you.
See you later, alligator.
After a while, crocodile.

Table of Contents

The Artist	xi
Section 1: PTSD and Trauma	**1**
Sadness	3
Carl Mobley	4
Paul	7
Silence	8
Section 2: Grief	**9**
The Little Girl	11
The Emotional Challenges of Grief	13
The Empty Chair	15
Christy Walsh	19
Deja Iwamoto	21
Emotional Confusion	22
The Whispers of the Vacant House	23
Section 3: Depression and Anxiety	**31**
Pacifying My Emotions	33
Oh, Loneliness	34
Ghost	36
The Raging Storm within Me	38
Everything Lost or Just Hidden by Hurt	40
The Lifeless, Misunderstood Tree	42
One Last Forgotten Teardrop	44

Section 4: Identity	**47**
My Ocean	49
Darren Jones	50
Tracy Steadman Henry	52
Do You See What I See?	54
The Seasons of My Mind	59
Who?	62
The Clamor of Anxiety	63
Flawed Intentions	64
Section 5: Life Choices and Strength	**65**
Thank You, Old, Rotting Tree Stump	67
Barry Stirbens	69
Giggles for Dad	71
What Is Love?	72
House	73
Oh, Dandelion	74
Oh, Weeping Willow Tree	75
Different Tree Named Me	77
Wings	79
Looking at Love	81
I Am Not Defined by PTSD, Trauma, Grief, Depression, or Anxiety	82

Captured in a second: one graceful, trickling teardrop.
Captured in a minute: a snapshot taken at that perfect moment.
Captured in an hour: solitude, staring at the stars in the sky.
Captured in a day: sadness for making an irreversible mistake.
Captured in a week: watching the snowbirds return.
Captured in a month: a new baby learning how to walk.
Captured in a year: life's moments of happiness and sadness.
Captured in a decade: raising children to become adults.
Captured in a century: grandparents seeing the world change spontaneously.
Captured in a lifetime: birth, a life full of events, passing down a legacy.

The Artist

The artist's tools are like magic
Paper
Pencils
Pens
Paint
Markers
Clay

Magic to an artist's mind
A pathway into a realm of imagination
A place that many people never find
Often misunderstood
Going out of the lines of reality

Pink clouds
Blue trees
Thin lines
Thick lines
Brushes of unique colors
Dotted figures

Sometimes only understood
By the artist
By the out-of-the-box thinker
By the believer of magic
Abstract

The artist's tools are like magic

Section 1

PTSD and Trauma

Sadness

Life is so sad when I feel like I'm really not in it.
I'm just a stranger looking from the outside in.
Pretending has become my presence.
Life is so sad when I feel like I'm not in it.

Carl Mobley

Vietnam War veteran
Enlisted at age eighteen
Interviewed on July 2, 2023

If you could capture how you felt when you enlisted in the army in 1966 to fight in the Vietnam War, what would you say?
I joined the army right out of high school. All my friends were joining to fight in the Vietnam War, and I didn't want to be left behind, so I joined in 1966. I was trained as a combat engineer and then was sent to fight immediately after that. When I was sent, I thought it was for a good cause.

If you could capture what you faced during the Vietnam War, what would you say?
We took care of the Vietcong I remember one time when we were given orders to evacuate a village that consisted of about one hundred houses. We then burned down the village. We were then told that it was the wrong village, and the military had to send in a construction company to rebuild the village.

We also were given orders that we were not allowed to fire on the enemy unless they fired on us. A lot of us disagreed with this and shot at anything that moved to protect our own lives and the lives of others. We played no games. It was all about staying alive and making it home to our families.

If you could capture what you faced when you came back home from the Vietnam War, what would you say?
When I got out and came home, I drove my motorcycle and didn't go home for two days. When I got home, I told my mom that if I was sleeping, then don't wake me up because I was still on edge from being in combat and that I would think she was the enemy. I had lots of trouble sleeping because of what I endured during the war. It didn't take much to make me jump up in my sleep to protect myself.

It was so hard to ease the painful memories of the war. I did go back to work as an engineer. I have been married four times. I couldn't settle down and get it together because of the flashbacks from the war. It took me six months to talk to people. It was as if I had crawled into a dark, deep hole. I had to take medications—and still do—because I have terrible dreams, and the medications help me to not remember the flashbacks. At the same time, asleep or awake, I knew that the flashbacks were there and that I was just going to have to learn to deal with them. A lot of times, I would take off alone and just look at nature.

If you could capture how the Vietnam War has affected you today, what would you say?
I still suffer from what I went through in Vietnam today. I worked for three years in the VA until I was diagnosed with congestive heart failure and had to stop working. I began to have too much time to think, and I started having bad flashbacks of my thoughts of Vietnam. I continue to deal with these flashbacks today because I have too much time on my hands to think about what happened during the war. I had to get help, so I went to the VA. I started group therapy.

Sometimes I would just sit there and listen to others and wouldn't say a word during the whole group session. I also saw a doctor there who helped me a lot. I had a horse for twenty-seven years and would go to the stables and talk to him every night. It was like he knew everything that I was saying. My horse was very comforting to me. I also have a service dog now, and he is my best friend. He lays at my feet. He is always with me. I can sum it up by saying my brain hones in on what happened during the war. If I keep thinking about it, my flashbacks just become bigger and bigger. It's like this: if you put your finger up and then put it down, do you forget it was up?

Paul

Vietnam War veteran
Drafted when he was eighteen years old
Interviewed on July 1, 2023

If you could capture how you felt to be drafted into the Vietnam War at the age of eighteen, what would you say?
I was afraid of leaving everyone behind and going to a hostile environment. I was also afraid of what was going to happen to me at such a young age.

If you could capture what you experienced during the war, what would you say?
I thought about whether I was going to make it home. I was in a remote environment with no working electricity or water for showers. We were given orders to not shoot unless shot at by the enemy. If I saw someone moving, I shot first to protect my life. I wasn't going to wait to get shot first.

If you could capture what it was like to return home from the war, what would you say?
It was hard for me to understand what the war was all about. It taught me to look at situations wholeheartedly for what they were worth and to continue with a strong heart, and things would get better tomorrow. The Vietnam War made me a stronger man. I went as a boy and came back as a man.

Silence

Silence,
From my heart.
Secrecy,
Of my emotions.
Safety,
From others' judgments.
Disillusioned,
That people will change.
Assurance,
That I am in control of hiding my emotions.
Silence,
What must be to protect my heart.

Section 2

Grief

The Little Girl

I once knew a little girl who thought she had *everything*.
Then she grew up and realized that she really had *nothing*.

The love in her heart was tainted by *darkness*
Fear began to haunt her and cover her with *sadness*.
Blue, once her favorite color, became her biggest *thunder*.
What she thought was *happiness* was just *sadness*.
She wished that she had never met *bad*.
Bad now made her very *mad*.

I once knew a little girl who thought she had *everything*.
Then she grew up and realized that she really had *nothing*.

The love in her heart was painted *dark purple*.
Happiness was a *midnight storm*.
Joy was just *hate*.
Feelings were *jaded* by hues of *dark blue*.

I once knew a little girl who thought she had *everything*.
Then she grew up and realized that she really had *nothing*.

Everything was about *midnight*.
Nothing was about *sunshine*.
Midnight overwhelmed her with lies,
Bringing dark rain clouds to her eyes.
The little happiness she did have in her life,
Was always jaded by *midnight*.

I once knew a little girl who thought she had *everything*.
Then she grew up and realized that she really had *nothing*.

Happiness began as a short, light summer breeze,
But quickly became a whirling *midnight freeze*.
The winds whirled and whirled.
The storm quietly sneaked in.
Violently, violently, violently!
Blurring everything ahead of her,
Blurring everything behind her,
Until *midnight* won.

I once knew a little girl who thought she had *everything*.
Then she grew up and realized that she only had *emptiness*.

The Emotional Challenges of Grief

Ralph Waldo Emerson wrote, "For each thorn, there's a rosebud...For each twilight—a dawn...For each trial—the strength to carry on, For each storm cloud—a rainbow...For each shadow—the sun...For each parting—sweet memories when sorrow is done."

I love this quote. Though it seems an oxymoron, Emerson shows us that for every dark tunnel that we travel through, eventually, there is a light at the end.

The emotional challenges of grief can weigh heavily on our hearts, turning our worlds upside down in the blink of an eye, and leaving us feeling like life will never be right side up again. I was very close to my grandparents, and when they passed away, the dark tunnel seemed endless. For a long time, I stayed there, thinking that there would never be a way out from the grief that I held in my heart.

Fortunately, over time, I have learned that grieving is perfectly normal, but at some point, we need to travel outside the darkness to the light. Then we can live in the present while still remembering the past and how it has affected us. Our stories are important and must be told. They will help with our healthy healing process and will also help those in our lives understand what we are going through so they can help us. Hopefully, the people in our lives will hear our message and remember it so they can pass it on to future generations.

I have grieved the loss of my grandparents and strive every day to live in the present while still cherishing the memories I had with them. This doesn't mean that I don't miss them anymore. In the present, I can still remember the things that I loved about them. In the future, I intend to carry on their legacy by telling stories about them to my children, grandchildren, and other generations. This seems easier said than done. Believe me, I still struggle with it today, but I am slowly finding my way out of the tunnel toward the light. It can be a long, slow process. Healing doesn't mean that we have forgotten the past. It just means we remember it and then we move on to the present while staying mindful and grounded.

The Empty Chair

I stare
From a distance
At the old, worn wooden rocking chair.
A woman
I once knew
Sat there.

She filled the chair
With laughter,
With silence,
With tears of joy,
With tears of sadness,
With a full heart,
With an empty heart.

I stare
From a distance
At the old, worn wooden rocking chair.
A woman
I once knew
Sat there.

Rocking and rocking
Her arms outstretched
Her lap always welcoming
Embracing anyone
With hope, love, comfort.

"Sit on my lap," she would say,
"Today, tomorrow, any day"

I stare
From a distance
At the old, worn wooden rocking chair.
A woman
I once knew
Sat there.

Rest your head on my shoulder.
Listen to my heartbeat
In rhythm with yours.
A faint beating heart,
Of past frightful memories.
A loud, drum like beating heart,
Full of joyful memories.

I stare
From a distance
At the old, worn wooden rocking chair.
A woman
I once knew
Sat there.

Her rocking
Always in rhythm
With her own heartbeat.
Rocking, rocking,
Faster and faster,
Thoughts of her own past happy memories.

Rocking, rocking,
Slower and slower,
Thoughts of her own past frightful memories.

I stare
From a distance
At my old, worn wooden rocking chair.
The woman
I knew so well
Sat there.

My rocking chair
Now only rocks with the wind.
Sitting empty,
Heartbroken,
No rhythm beats from it.
Only a deafening silence
No happiness
No sadness.

Yesterday
Today
Or any day.

I stare
One last time
From a distance
At the old, worn wooden rocking chair.
A woman
I once knew
Sat there.

Seeing the shadow of the woman
That I can only see.
She rocks and rocks
Until she rocks no more.
Getting up
She runs her fingers
Over each part of that old, wooden rocking chair.
And then slowly turns away

I stare
One last time
From a distance
At the old
Worn
Wooden
Rocking chair.
A woman
I once knew
Sat there.

Christy Walsh

The future is no more uncertain than the present.
—Walt Whitman

Grieving the loss of a child
Interviewed on July 1, 2023

If you could capture in a moment how the loss of your child has affected you, what would you say?
With the loss of my daughter, the emptiness and the feelings of hopelessness became my home. I faced this depression on a daily basis. My depression was like a black hole in which I had lost myself.

If you could capture in a moment what you experienced during the grieving process, what would you say?
It was a challenge finding people to talk to about how I felt. I had to go to a grieving help group to be supported by people who went through what I went through.

If you could capture in a moment what you faced when you had to return to a somewhat normal day-to-day life without your child, what would you say?
I was forced into returning to a normal life. I was drinking and crying all the time. Then I got pregnant and had to get sober again for my newborn baby.

If you could capture in a moment how the loss of your child has affected you today, what would you say?
She is still constantly living in my life even though she is not with me. The anniversary of her death, her birthday, her siblings not having her around—I constantly think about what she would have looked like at her age and what she would be doing. These things are constant reminders that she is not here, but I can't dwell on it. I had to move on.

Deja Iwamoto

Grieving the loss of a grandmother at fourteen years old
Interviewed on July 6, 2023

If you could capture in a moment how you felt from the loss of your grandmother when you were fourteen years old, what would you say?
I was sad because she was my best friend. I missed not having a best friend like her.

If you could capture in a moment the struggles that you faced during the grieving process, what would you say?
I kept to myself. I was lonely. I missed her because she was my best friend. I always helped her.

If you could capture in a moment how losing your grandmother has affected you today, what would you say?
It was weird because I was used to helping her and being with her. I hadn't gotten over it yet, but I had to move on. I put on a smile every day so that people thought I was OK.

Emotional Confusion

One day my world
Upside down.
Another day
My world
Right side up.
Other days my world
A combination
Upside down
Right side up.

The Whispers of the Vacant House

I sit hesitantly in my Volkswagen Beetle.
I have sat in this driveway
A million times or so.

Staring at your house
Holding my steering wheel
So tightly
Reddish-purple hands
Hesitant to go inside
Oh, vacant house.

Your whispers, whispers,
Beckoning me to come inside.
So I whisper back,
I will visit you one last time.

Oh, vacant house
You then whisper to me,
I am all alone now.
I miss you.
Without you
My walls have
No beginnings
No endings.

I release my hands
Open my car door
Stand up

Knees wobbly
Hands shaky
Shallow breathing
Heart beating
Faster and faster
As I am drawn
To your side door
Oh, vacant house.

I see you
Oh, vacant house
Just as you are.
Inhaling
Exhaling
Inhaling
Exhaling
With each whisper.
Your screen door
Opens with a strong gust of wind.
Your door is unlocked.
Did you unlock it for me?

I hesitantly open you.
I follow your whispers.
My heart flutters.
As I walk inside
Tears stream down my face.
My heart beats
Louder, louder, louder.

The four walls of your kitchen
Look the same,

But something is missing.
Feelings of emptiness
Well up inside me.

Oh, vacant house
Once
Full of
Kisses,
Joyfulness,
Tears,
Laughter,
Silliness,
Family voices.

No candy jar on the counter.
I remember you
As a child
As an adult.
Always filled
With red cinnamon candy,
Green and white spearmint candy,
More candy than I can remember.

My hands went into you
Like catching a goldfish in a bowl.
Getting one favorite piece of candy,
Then sneaking two or three more.
Grandma's
Candy jar full.

The white-speckled kitchen table
Three grandchildren once sat.

Breakfast
Set for what felt like queens.
A white coffee cup
Waiting to have hot chocolate.
Cereal...toast...
Oh, and Grandpa's shredded wheat
With hot water poured over it.
At that same, white-speckled table
We once played Skip-Bo and Uno.

I walk into the living room,
Grandpa's clowns
Once in a display cabinet.
No clowns now
No display cabinet.

A blue plush recliner
Grandpa read
National Geographic.
Gone
Except for the indents in the carpet.

The pullout sleeper sofa
Three ornery grandchildren
Raised chaos during sleepovers.

The family pictures on the walls
My mom and dad
My uncle and aunt
Me, my sister, and three cousins.
The grandfather clock

Beating like a drum.
Ding-dong, ding-dong.

Grandma and Grandpa's bedroom
I was always so excited to go in there.
Grandpa gave us little surprises.
Canadian money
I collected each piece.
It was like gold to me.
A half of a stick of gum.
I still wonder,
Why only Canadian money?
Why only half a stick of gum?

The back family room
Grandma's puzzles and paintings.
She wore a flashlight band
Like a coal miner,
Her eyes growing old.
Perfection in each puzzle
Perfection in each painting

A television
The Idiot Box
Grandma and Grandpa
Lawrence Welk
Choice of soda
With a straw.
The popcorn machine
Saturday night sleepovers

The enclosed porch
Now empty
No furniture.
Grandma's green thumb
Displayed inside this room
Beautiful Christmas cacti

As I sit on your carpet
For the last time,
Staring out of the porch
Glass windows,
Still surrounded with beauty.
Picturesque green grass
Once Grandpa's Garden
Now gone.

I hear your whispers
Oh, vacant house.
Gazing again
I remember
Beautiful multicolored flowers
A luscious garden
Potatoes
Tomatoes
Cucumbers
Lettuce
Green beans
Green peppers
Carrots

Oh, and I can't forget
Grandpa

Wearing that silly garden hat
Blue jeans with visible holes
A white T-shirt
A dress shirt
Sleeves rolled up
Black socks
White tennis shoes.
A gardener he looked like.
A gardener he was.
His thumb,
Greener than I have ever seen.

Oh, vacant house
Once
Full of
Kisses
Joyfulness
Tears
Laughter
Silliness
Family voices.

Oh, vacant house
You then whisper to me,
I am all alone now.
I miss you.
Without you
My walls have
No beginnings
No endings...

But that is not true
Oh, vacant house.
I whisper to you,
You are not alone.
No walls, beginnings, endings
To the human eye,
But to me
Your beginnings and endings
Forever imprinted
Memories

Section 3

Depression and Anxiety

Pacifying My Emotions

I wear my heart of depression and anxiety in a place deep within my soul. On the outside I wear my face with a smile. Hopefully, nobody sees my pain.
—Tracy Henry

I struggle with anxiety and depression. My diagnosis frequently makes me feel like I live in two different worlds. My emotions feel so out of control that daylight seems to never come, and darkness endlessly traps me. Social norms cause people to think of me as crazy, out of control, and not to be trusted. Sometimes, I really don't know who I think I am. Could I be the person they think I am? Maybe not?

> Dear Self,
> I know that you will be disappointed in me by the time I finish this note. You see, you have never been my best friend or even an acquaintance. I know that you don't like to hear me talking about you this way, but I am just trying to be honest with you and let you know how I really feel.
>
> Sincerely,
> Self

Oh, Loneliness

Oh, Loneliness
Please stop calling my name,
Your best friend, Depression
Can do the same.

Oh, Loneliness
You cloud my brain
With nothingness.
Your best friend, Depression
Makes Loneliness feel like my best friend.

Oh, Loneliness
Let's have a heart-to-heart talk
Because you are ruining my life
Shutting down
My feelings
My emotions
My will to live.

Oh, Depression
You think you know me
But you don't.
I know that you try to make me feel nothingness,
But I know nothingness too well.
You can't fool me with your spell.

Nothingness
I think you are the sensible one
Because nothingness feels like nothing.
No more sadness,
No more worries,
No more lies,
No more crying.

Somethingness
Expressions
Sadness
Worries
Crying.

Expressions
Everyone has them
Perfectly normal
Expressions.

Nothingness
Somethingness
Who will take over?
Somethingness,
I hope
You will become
My best friend
In the end.

Ghost

I feel like a ghost
Am I really one?
Floating above
Lots of people
I drift around
A crowd of people
Not really understanding anything.
I say
They say
It makes me sad.
It makes me mad.
It makes me paranoid.
The ghost I have become.

When I look in the mirror
Ugliness I see.
My ears, eyes, and mouth
Contorted

Paranoid to be around anyone
Fear overtakes me
Will I say the wrong thing?
Will I do the wrong thing?
I get there and instantly say
"Let's get out of here."

Impulsivity overtakes me
So I become a ghost
Sometimes not even saying goodbye.

Being a ghost
No one to judge me,
No one to whisper about me,
No one to ridicule me,
Just me
A ghost

The Raging Storm within Me

If you are coping with depression, sometimes depression is actually anger turned inward.
—Stephanie Moulton Sarkis, PhD

Depression, for me, is like climbing the walls of a cave. During my deepest states, it takes over me. I feel like I, and only I, can claw my way out of the cave to reach the light above. I can only do this by using my fingernails on its dark, steep sides. Unfortunately, sometimes, my fingernails are jagged and broken, unable to adequately claw up the sides. I am left with cuts, sores, and trickling blood on my fingers and hands that eventually become scares that remind me daily of my darkest depression. Sometimes, my depression is short-lived and easier to climb out of. No matter what kind of depression I am going through, it always clouds my thoughts for varying amounts of time. I feel like I am entranced in what feels like a state of confusion because of its timelessness and endlessness.

My depression is an indescribable silence. I feel like a puppet lying in a dark box, untouched by human life for what seems like forever. Am I even still alive? I can't move my arms or legs. My mouth feels like it is glued shut, making it impossible to. I scream for help. My eyes see nothing but darkness. Have I been forgotten? Have I just lost my own identity to reality?

My depression is a place where I am taken to for protection from my enslaved emotions, a quiet place that draws me into a deep sleep in the nothingness of my life's turbulence.

My emotions are sucked into the vortex of my storm. The silence here is as quiet as the sound of a pin dropping on the floor. The area right outside the vortex is still a turbulent storm of emotions that spin around and around in my mind, leaving me with little control to get out of this dreamlike state.

My anger at the unpredictability of my life and reality is sucked into the eye of the storm, only to be imprisoned by its rapture which is in a state of confusion. When my anger can rest, I am startled out of what feels like a deep sleep. When I do come out of this deep sleep, I am always hypersensitive to everything: the warmth of the sun on my face, the blinding brightness to my eyes, the sound of rustling leaves in the trees, the sweet smell of roses, the succulent taste of sweet honeysuckle.

I now know that this depression will come and go. It will be something that I always struggle with. The fight for survival is not over; depression is my forever reality. Learning to cope with it will always be an everyday struggle for me.

The realization that I have depression is the first step in learning to cope with it. I now know that when I was in the cave, trying to climb by myself, I could have yelled out for help. Someone would likely have heard my cries and helped me. They might have bungee jumped down into the cave to bring me back to the light. They might have also thrown a rope down for me to climb my way up. It might have been harder, but the struggle is worth the fight. Hopefully, there will be more days of light than darkness. Fight, fight, fight. Never give up.

Everything Lost or Just Hidden by Hurt

Every moment lost
From them?
From me?

Hurtful words said
By them?
By me?

Drips of blood
Still found on
Their hearts?
My heart?

Hellos, goodbyes
From them?
From me?
From myself?

Distance created
From them?
From me?
From myself?

Regrets past
From them?
From me?
From myself?

Unconditional love
Not from them
Not for myself.

When the time comes
Under my control
With my guard taken down
I will feel at peace.

Envisioning myself
Lying in a beautiful field
Of vibrant, colored flowers,
I make the decision
Refusing to not stand lifeless.

Trying everything to exist
Through
Highs
Lows.
Keep fighting
Unconditionally
For myself
Because
I deserve it.

The Lifeless, Misunderstood Tree

In the forest
A multitude of trees
Waking up in spring
Full of life.
Blooming flowers
In vibrant colors
Reds, yellows, greens, lavenders.

In the same forest
A once living tree
Not waking up in spring,
No blooming flowers
No vibrant colors.

Just a barren tree
A limp, dry tree
Alone in the forest
Surrounded
Hidden
By all the living trees.

If the lifeless tree is found
It may be too late.
Snapped, dry branches
Stepped on
Used for firewood
Long misunderstood.

The living trees
Turning their backs
Enjoying their own beauty
Making a loud, sweet melody
Ignoring the lifeless tree.

One Last Forgotten Teardrop

My heart
Beating
Blood pumping
In, out, in, out
Slower, slower, slower
Filled with
Hate?
Abandonment?
Fear?
Resentment?
Unloved?
Untouched?

Memories
Lost?
Buried?
Covered forever?
Why?
I can't remember
Or did you even exist?

My face
No eyes
No ears
No nose
No mouth
Nonexistence

My hands
Blue
Frostbitten
Missing fingers
Untouchable
Full of pain

My feet
Bare
Calloused
Full of thorns
Walking, walking
Where?

Nothingness is lonely
I am disappearing
Ever so slowly

Will I blow away
As a gust of wind
Engulfed with sand
Never remembered?

I am
One last forgotten
Teardrop

I wear my heart of depression and anxiety in a place deep within my soul. On the outside I wear my face with a smile. Hopefully nobody sees my pain.

Section 4

Identity

My Ocean

Never underestimate the intentions of others.
—Tracy Steadman Henry

My ocean has no beginning and no ending. I have little control over my waves that rush in and out, in and out. A variety of creatures live within me. At any given time, hidden under or above me, there may be so many things going on that many people would go bonkers trying to take it all in. What people see above the waves is my anxiety, depression, and more. But my waves have eccentric life below my surface: blue goldfish, whales, and sharks of different sizes and shapes, along with multicolored plants of green, orange, yellow, and turquoise. These sights put me in a trancelike state.

I stare at the glow of the full moon in the clear skies above me. Stars painted and scattered everywhere in the sky exhilarate me. My waves titillate me in such a way that I become alive. My waves move back and forth, back and forth. My waves are filled with the sound of whoosh-whoosh, whoosh-whoosh. The saltiness of my water makes me thirst for more, and more, and more. Waves tickle me in the sand on the beach, making me giggle with pure excitement. My unique smell may be pungent to some but delectable to others. This is my ocean and only my ocean. When you come to me, please respect my inner and outer beauty, just as I would respect the beauty of your ocean.

Darren Jones

Facing mental and physical health challenges
Interviewed on February 23, 2024

If you could capture your thoughts and feelings about having mental health and physical health diagnoses what would you tell people?
Having mental and physical health problems has been difficult and good at the same time. I became a stronger person after my heart surgery in 2008.

If you could capture the challenges that you face daily, what would you tell people?
I don't like working alone. I need a routine for work and home. A routine is very important to me.

If you could capture the challenges that you face daily to try to fit into society, what would you tell people?
I have always been a loner, especially during high school. I was bullied a lot. As an adult, I try to just fit in, and most of the time it works. I try to just be myself. If people try to bully me, I try to just ignore them.

If you could capture how these challenges have affected you today, what would you say? What would you tell people if they asked you how your mental health and physical health challenges have affected you today?

Because of my heart issues, I am on a blood thinner. This blood thinner prevents me from participating in contact sports and from weightlifting. I basically can only exercise by walking.

Tracy Steadman Henry

Facing mental health challenges
July 6, 2023

If you could capture your thoughts and feelings about having a mental health diagnosis, what would you tell people?
Facing my mental health challenges made me feel so lost in myself—like I was screaming for help deep within my soul, and no matter how hard I tried, I couldn't get the screaming to stop or at least come out.

If you could capture the challenges that you face daily, what would you tell people?
Living with a mental health diagnosis is a daily challenge, and I have to deal with the ups and downs of that day. Some days I wake up and I feel exuberant and on top of the world. Other days I wake up in a fog, wondering how I am going to make it through the day. And still other days I wake up exuberant and then somewhere in the day I crash, causing my depression to kick in. Either way anxiety is an everyday thing for me.

If you could capture the challenges that you face daily to try to fit into society, what would you tell people?
I was and still am trying to figure out what the word "normal" means. What qualities define a person who is normal? What standards define a world that is normal? I found a caring psychiatrist that I see monthly or more often if needed. She is knowledgeable and caring. She listens to me, and

together we figure out what the best treatment is for me. I also see a caring and knowledgeable therapist, and during each session I talk about what I am feeling. She helps me to continue to learn coping skills that I can use in my day-to-day life. I could say that I have it all figured out, but I don't. I am going to always have anxiety and depression, and I know that I will have to battle my way up during the low days and enjoy the good days.

If you could capture how these challenges have affected you today, what would you say? What would you tell people if they asked you how your mental health challenges have affected you today?

I am challenged every day to understand who I was, who I am now, and who I want to be. Mental health challenges are just that: *challenges*. I might wake up one day and think it is going to be a great day, and then slowly it becomes a lonely day. Emotions, realities, a sense of self, and a sense of others' intentions are just some of the ways that different mental challenges have affected me today. Life is different for me, and I have accepted this. Finding a way to understand myself and be understood by others is the greatest challenge that I face.

Do You See What I See?

When you look at me
Do you see what I see?

You see a woman
With a smile on her face.

I see a different woman
Concealing sadness.

You see a woman
Covered in tattoos.
Staring
You look away.

I see a different woman
Covered in tattoos.
Her life story
For all to see.

You see a woman
All put together.

You see a woman
Giving,
Humble.

I see a woman
Never giving to herself.
A wilted flower inside
Forgotten,
Unwatered.

You see a woman
Talking to everyone
Free-spirited,
Funny.

I see a woman
Talking to everyone
Only to hide her anxieties.

You see a woman
Lighthearted
Quite contagious.

I see a woman
Heavyhearted
Hurt
Never-ending.

You see a woman
Strong
Full of pride.

I see a woman
Weak
Secretly hidden.

You see a woman
Never shedding a tear.

I see a woman
Hidden tears
A broken heart.

You see a woman
Intelligent
All put together.

I see a woman
With impulsive racing thoughts
Haunting me
Night and day.

You see a woman
Full of words
That flutter
Off her tongue
Like the wings
Of a beautiful butterfly.

I see a woman
Tongue-tied
Annoying to many.

You see a woman
The perfect mom.

I see a woman
A heart
Broken into pieces
By her own doing
By others' too.

You see a woman
Never feeling alone
In a room full of people.

I see a woman
So very alone
Invisible
To a room full of people.

You see a woman
A gardener
Tending to beautiful flowers.

I see a woman
Ugly weeds
Strangling.

You see a woman
Daring.

I see a woman
Afraid to go outside.

You see a woman
Overabundance of giving.

I see a woman
Empty
With nothing more to give.

You see a woman.
I see another woman.

The Seasons of My Mind

Spring, summer, fall, winter
Filling my mind
Some days all of you
Some days three of you
Some days two of you
Some days one of you
Some days none of you.

Spring, summer, fall, winter
No matter the days
No matter the *season*
In my mind
I can find no reason
You just exist.

The spell of fall
My mind
Like in a spell
Floating, falling
Multicolored leaves
A true trickery of my mind?
Who was I?
Green?
Who am I now?
Red? Orange? Yellow?
Who will I be?
Blue?
Fall.

Spring, summer, fall, winter
No matter the days
No matter the *seasons*
In my mind
I can find no reason
You just exist.

Captured by winter
Like a winter storm
Confusion?
Whirling
This way
That way
Delusions of my mind?
Winter.

Spring, summer, fall, winter
No matter the days
No matter the *season*
In my mind
I can find no reason
You just exist.

Did I hear you, spring?
A din in my right ear?
Children outside loudly
Stomping, stomping, stomping!
A din in my left ear?
Neighbors outside loudly
Talking, talking, talking!

A din in both ears?
Stomping! Talking! Stomping! Talking!
Spring.

Spring, summer, fall, winter
No matter the days
No matter the *seasons*
In my mind
I now find a reason
Your beauty exists.

Summer, is that you?
Sunflowers
Sundial
Perceptive bees
Perpetual winds
Scarlet strawberries
Like a beautiful rose of red
Summer.

Spring, summer, fall, winter
No matter the days
No matter the *seasons*
In my mind
I now find a reason
Your beauty exists.

Who?

Who am I now?
Who was I before?
Who will I become?

Who are they now?
Who were they before?
Who will they become?

Will they hurt me now?
Did they hurt me before?
Will they hurt me again?

The Clamor of Anxiety

Clamor
In my heart
Noise
Stirred-up emotions
Vulnerability
Opening my bleeding heart
Enthusiastic
Understanding
Denial
Brushing off untruths
Clamor

Flawed Intentions

Often, I get so self-absorbed that I question the intentions of the people I come in contact with from day to day. For instance, I might come in contact with a retail worker who seems irritated and short with me. In such moments, I may assume that she is always irritated and short with customers when she may have been up all night with a sick baby. My anxiety can cause me to be so impulsive in what I say and do, leading me to vocalize thoughts such as, "What's her problem? Good customer service should be expected by every worker all the time." Consequently, I might go to a different checkout lane the next time I am in the store to avoid dealing with her ever again.

In today's society, we are so self-absorbed regarding others' intentions toward us that we forget to look at our own intentions toward them. I know I have flaws. Everyone has flaws.

Like the lady in the retail store, I'm sure she didn't get up that morning and think, "I am going to have bad intentions today. I am going to be irritated and short with people." After all, people don't wake up each morning and know what the day will be like for them. Just as we have imperfections, so do others.

My point is to know that everyone has bad and good intentions, but at the same time, no human being is perfect. Give yourself a break when you make a mistake. Get back up and keep trying. Don't let your anxieties take over in how you act and what you say. Impulsivity can be so very poisonous to yourself and to others. Once something is said or done, it is hard to undo it.

Section 5

Life Choices and Strength

Thank You, Old, Rotting Tree Stump

If you have never failed you have never lived.
—Abraham Lincoln

I saw an old, rotting tree stump
At the end of the forest.
What had you once been?
A sturdy tree?
Maybe king of the forest?

I went over
Wanting to sit on you
But hesitant
Your outsides
Brittle
Deteriorated
Scattered pieces.

I decide to sit on you
With gentleness.
Will you fall apart?
To my surprise
Sturdy and strong
Hidden inner strength.

My eyes
Full of tears
Fall down my cheeks.
Maybe

Just maybe
People will not judge me
By my outward appearance
But instead take the time
To sit with me for a while.

Know me on the inside
My beating heart.
My compassionate soul
My feelings.

Thank you old, rotting tree stump
For giving me the strength to sit on you.

Barry Stirbens

The life challenges of blindness
Interviewed December 10, 2023

If you could capture in a moment how blindness has affected you, what would you say?
First, blindness has affected my relationships with people in a positive sense. As a minister I can relate to people who are struggling with something that they are facing by empathizing and sympathizing with where they are at. I have also used my blindness to help teach people that no matter what your circumstances are, you can be successful by just being who you are.

Second, I don't relate to sight and the environment around me, so I rely on my other senses.

If you could capture in a moment some of the things that you have had to adapt to in your day-to-day life, what would you say?
It took me longer to do my sermon preparations. For pastoral calls, I had to find someone to take me. Braille on cans and foods, knowing where things were and keeping them in the same location, and keeping clothing in a special place in the closet. I can identify most things by how they feel. If I had a funeral, wedding, or other special events, things would be put in a special place.

If you could capture in a moment how you could use your experiences of being blind to help other people, what would you say?
I would reach out and talk to these individuals about reading services, audio services with mobility and getting around, and societies such as the Philanthropy Society. People who are blind are very good at helping other people who are blind by giving them advice and direction.

Giggles for Dad

My dad is so silly.
I like when he tickles me.
I giggle and jump in my bed.
Tickle
Giggle
Tickle
Giggle
I am out of breath.
Stop, Dad, stop!
Tickle
Giggle
Tickle
Giggle

What Is Love?

Lovebirds singing
The glowing of the moon
The warmth of the morning sunrise
The beauty of the sunset
Watching that one special shooting star
Lovers holding hands
Kissing in the park
A light breeze blowing in the wind
Little children laughing and playing
A new beginning
A lifetime of memories
Love

House

Once
Shipwrecked
Now
Salvaged
Once
Weather-beaten
Now
Sophisticated
Once
Voiceless
Now
Chatty
Once
Dingy
Now
Immaculate
Once
Unloved
Now
Endearing
Once
Old
Now
Made anew

Oh, Dandelion

Oh, dandelion
With your veined stem
Conspicuously overtaking
Luscious green grasses

Oh, dandelion
With your lone yellow
Grotesquely oversized
Soon limp and withered
Human hands
Incompetent *weed*

Oh, dandelion
With your strong green stem
Ambitiously
Sprouting
Hues of green

Oh, dandelion
With your radiant shades of yellow
Luminous to the human eye
Little girls' and boys' hands
Gently picking you
True *flower* of love

Oh, Weeping Willow Tree

The future is no more uncertain than the present.
—Walt Whitman

Oh, weeping willow tree
I remember you so vividly
As a child
With your drooping
Branches
Leaves
Hanging so low
As if holding
My sadness
My insecurities

Oh, weeping willow tree
I remember you so well
As a child
I hid under you
Crying my tears
Like the rain
That rushes down your leaves

Oh, weeping willow tree
I knew you so well
As a child
We only knew
The sadness
I held in my heart

The secrets
I hid underneath your shadows
From others
From myself

Oh, weeping willow tree
I remember you differently now
As an adult
I notice your sturdy trunk
My past and present
Etched upon your bark
For everyone to see

Different Tree Named Me

I've always thought
That trees were just trees
What else could they be?

But trees are not just trees.
They are all different.
Different names
Different scents
Different colors
Different purposes
Witnesses to life or death

I've always thought
That people were just people
Trees were just trees
What else could they be?

But people are not just people.
They are all different.
Different names
Different scents
Different colors
Different purposes
Life and death

I've always thought
That people were just people
What else could they be?

The birth of new trees
Share the same heartbeat of *life*
Trees of longevity
The death of old trees
Not able to stand anymore
Share the same heartbeat of life
Both part of the soil that birthed them

I've always thought
Trees were just trees.
People were just people.
They are all different.
I can be me
Whatever that may be
And you can be you!

Wings

The sky
Painted
Light blue
Clouds
White streaks
Fluffy cotton balls
Translucent

A hawk
Wings
Spotted
A reddish hue
Spreading
Indefinitely
Soaring
Strength
Holding
A stocky build

The hawk
Each day comes
Descending lower and lower
Then soaring higher and higher

Tempting me
Spreading
My wings
Soaring

Higher and higher
Lower and lower

Trusting
My wings
Of strength
To carry my heavy load
Freedom, freedom, freedom

At last!

Looking at Love

Love is the whole thing. We are only pieces.
—Rumi

Love recognizes no barriers.
—Maya Angelou

'Tis better to have loved and lost than never to have loved at all.
—Alfred Lord Tennyson

We love the things we love for what they are.
—Robert Frost

I Am Not Defined by PTSD, Trauma, Grief, Depression, or Anxiety

I am a compassionate person.
I am a published author.
I am a teacher.
I am an artist.
I am a storyteller.
I am a soprano.
I am a pianist

My tattoos tell the story of my life.
I color outside of the lines.

I love sports cars.
I love memoirs.
I love dragonflies.
I love butterflies.
I love the color lavender.
I love genealogy.
I love silly hair.
I love nature.
I love Mexican petunias.
I love sports.
I love Volkswagen Beetles.
I love chimpanzees.
I love walks on the beach.

I am not defined by PTSD, trauma, grief, depression, or anxiety.

About the Author

Tracy Steadman Henry, a retired educator, is a distinguished author known for her debut book, The Little Girl Who Survived the Great Depression, published in 2017. Her teaching career was marked by the prestigious Teacher of the Year award. Tracy's writings are inspired by her experiences and the joy she finds in her family, which includes three children, seven grandchildren, and her beloved dog, Phoebe. Her latest work, *Captured*, is a testament to her empathetic understanding of mental and physical health challenges, offering readers a profound insight into the experiences of those living with these conditions.

www.ingramcontent.com/pod-product-compliance
Lightning Source LLC
LaVergne TN
LVHW092056060526
838201LV00047B/1415